Table of Contents

1 Introduction to Jargon

Understanding jargon isn't simply about memorizing words; it's about grasping the underlying concepts they represent. Each field possesses its own unique vocabulary, a specialized language developed over time to facilitate efficient communication among its practitioners. This shared understanding, however, often creates an exclusionary barrier for those outside the specific domain. Imagine attending a medical conference without understanding terms like "hematoma" or "angiogenesis." You'd feel lost, unable to participate fully in discussions and presentations. This is the power, and the problem, of jargon.

The effective use of jargon hinges on context. Within a group of experts, its use speeds up communication, enhancing efficiency and precision. Think of surgeons swiftly exchanging information during an operation. The precise terminology allows for immediate understanding and action, critical in high-pressure situations. Conversely, using specialized language with a less knowledgeable audience can lead to confusion, misinformation, or even mistrust. A doctor explaining a complex medical condition to a patient needs to carefully select their words, explaining concepts without resorting to jargon that could alienate or worry the patient. The goal is always clarity, not obfuscation.

Therefore, mastering jargon is not just about knowing the terms but also understanding when and how to use them effectively.
Consider the legal profession. A lawyer's understanding of "habeas corpus," "stare decisis," or "voir dire" is paramount. These terms are the building blocks of their practice, allowing them to precisely articulate legal arguments and navigate complex procedures. Similarly, financial experts navigate the world of "hedge funds," "derivatives," and "capital gains" with ease. These are essential terms for them, part of the professional vernacular used to conduct business. But what about individuals who are not part of these disciplines? They need accessible explanations that translate the jargon into readily understandable language. Effective communication bridges this gap.
This requires a deliberate shift in perspective. Instead of viewing jargon as an inherent good or evil, consider it a tool – a powerful one, capable of great precision, but also potentially prone to misuse. Therefore, successful navigation of jargon requires a combination of vocabulary acquisition and context-sensitive application. Simply memorizing a list of terms isn't sufficient; understanding the conceptual underpinnings is crucial. Think about learning a new language; it's not just about translating words but understanding the cultural nuances associated with them. Jargon functions in a similar manner, incorporating cultural aspects specific to its discipline.
The best approach to learning jargon involves active engagement, not passive memorization. Immerse yourself in the field, reading relevant literature, listening to discussions, and asking questions. Engage with experts and seek clarifications when needed. This active process promotes deeper understanding, making the acquisition of specialized lan-

guage more meaningful and useful. Don't be afraid to ask for explanations; clarifying ambiguous terms demonstrates initiative and a willingness to learn, aspects appreciated within any professional community. Ultimately, your goal is not simply to understand jargon but to utilize it purposefully, applying it in a way that enhances communication and fosters understanding in diverse settings.

Furthermore, effective communication transcends the mere understanding of specialized terminology. It involves clarity of expression, logical presentation, and the ability to adapt your language to your audience. Consider the difference between a scientific paper and a popular science article; both may deal with the same subject matter, but their language dramatically differs to suit the knowledge level of the readers. This adaptability is paramount; it reflects a sophisticated understanding of the use of jargon, demonstrating the ability to tailor communication to specific audiences.

Learning jargon should not be an intimidating process. Instead, view it as an enriching opportunity to understand and engage more effectively with different professions. Through active learning, targeted reading, and a willingness to participate, you can successfully navigate this intricate world, transforming what may initially seem like an impenetrable maze into a navigable landscape. Ultimately, you should aim to use jargon effectively, only when appropriate and with a sensitivity toward your audience's comprehension level. This approach will show that your knowledge goes beyond simply memorizing terms.

Finally, remember that the field of jargon itself is dynamic. New terms continually emerge, reflecting advancements and changes in respective fields. This constant evolution highlights the importance of continuous learning, embracing the ongoing need to adapt and update your knowledge base. Staying current with new developments within your professional circles and staying informed about emerging language practices will ensure that your comprehension of jargon remains sharp and relevant, allowing for a more efficient and precise communication with others in your profession. The effective use of specialized terms, applied appropriately and thoughtfully, significantly enhances your overall communication skills.

1.1 What is Jargon?

Jargon, at its core, is specialized language used within a particular group or profession. It's a shorthand, a form of efficient communication among those who share a common understanding. Think of doctors discussing a patient's "tachycardia" – they understand it instantly as a rapid heart rate; a layman might need a lengthy explanation. This inherent efficiency, however, often comes at a cost. The same specialized terms that accelerate communication among insiders can easily exclude and confuse outsiders. This creates a barrier to understanding, hindering clear communication and potentially causing misunderstandings, especially in situations requiring collaboration between specialists and non-specialists. Therefore, understanding jargon's dual nature – its utility and its potential for exclusion – is crucial.

Consider the legal field, a realm teeming with Latin terms and complex phrasing. A contract's "force majeure" clause, for instance, signifies an unforeseen event that relieves a party from its contractual obligations. While lawyers readily understand this, explaining it to a non-legal audience requires careful unpacking and simplification. Similarly, in finance, terms like "derivatives" or "hedge funds" can be daunting even to those with a basic understanding of financial markets. These specialized terms represent complex financial instruments and investment strategies, requiring in-depth knowledge to fully grasp their meaning and implications. This inherent complexity often requires significant study and experience.

The challenge with jargon isn't always about the terms themselves; it's frequently about the context and the assumptions made by the speaker or writer. Assuming shared knowledge that doesn't exist can lead to significant communication breakdowns. A scientist might casually mention a "double-blind study," a standard research methodology, without realizing that a non-scientist may not understand its core elements – namely, the random assignment of participants to treatment and control groups, as well as the masking of both participants and researchers to the treatment assignments, to minimize bias. The intent isn't to deliberately obfuscate; it's simply the unconscious use of language reflective of one's professional world.

Effective communication transcends the use of jargon. While it might offer expediency within a particular professional community, its widespread use demands conscious consideration of the audience. Using jargon in presentations to a mixed audience, for example, demonstrates a lack of audience awareness and potentially alienates those lacking specialized knowledge. This might hinder understanding and reduce the effectiveness of the communication, making it a less than optimal choice. The solution involves a clear understanding of both the audience and the topic at hand.

Therefore, mastering communication involves more than simply memorizing specialized terms. It requires the ability to adapt language to the audience. A seasoned professional should be able to effortlessly switch between precise jargon when conversing with colleagues and clear, concise language when addressing a broader audience. This adaptability is a cornerstone of effective communication, ensuring information reaches its intended audience regardless of their level of familiarity with the subject matter. Understanding jargon's intricacies is not merely about recognizing specialized terms; it's about appreciating its power and its potential pitfalls, and using that understanding to foster clearer, more inclusive communication. It's about bridging the gap between specialized knowledge and wider understanding. The ability to communicate effectively across audiences is a skill essential for professionals in any field. The judicious use of jargon enhances communication, while its misuse creates obstacles to shared understanding. Developing this skill means consciously choosing the right words for each specific audience and situation.

It's not simply about avoiding jargon altogether; rather, it's about using it judiciously and strategically. Introducing a new term and then immediately providing a clear, non-jargon explanation is an effective strategy. For instance, one might introduce the term "epidemiology" and immediately follow with its simple definition: the study of the patterns, causes, and effects of health and disease in defined populations. This approach aids comprehension and ensures that the communication remains accessible to all. This mindful approach shows a conscious effort to build a shared understanding, enhancing the overall communication process.

Beyond simply defining terms, it is equally crucial to understand the nuances of jargon in its context. One term can mean entirely different things within different fields. For example, "resolution" can refer to the sharpness of an image in photography, the clarity of a legal matter in law, or the conclusion of a conflict in diplomacy. Understanding the context is key to avoiding misinterpretations and promoting clarity, and is crucial for understanding jargon. The same word can take on many layers of meaning; the key to understanding rests in the context in which it's used.

Learning to decipher jargon involves actively seeking out explanations and definitions, engaging with professional literature and utilizing resources like dictionaries and glossaries specific to your field. It's a continuous learning process, requiring diligent effort and a willingness to constantly expand your vocabulary. It also involves asking clarifying questions when encountering unfamiliar terms—demonstrating a commitment to understanding and fostering a more collaborative and inclusive environment. Proactive engagement is crucial to mastering jargon in any given field. It is a journey, not a destination.

Ultimately, navigating the jungle of jargon requires mindful consideration of both its benefits and its pitfalls. It is a tool, powerful in the right hands, but dangerous when wielded carelessly. By consciously choosing appropriate language for different audiences and by actively seeking to bridge the gap between specialized knowledge and general understanding, professionals can harness the efficiency of jargon without sacrificing clarity and inclusivity. Mastering jargon demands a delicate balance—efficient communication within specialized circles, and effective communication to broader audiences. It's a skill essential for anyone seeking to master their field and share its knowledge with others.

1.2 Why Jargon Matters

Effective communication hinges on shared understanding, and that's where jargon's double-edged sword comes into play. While it fosters efficient communication among specialists, its exclusionary nature can create significant barriers for those outside the immediate field. Consider a medical professional discussing a patient's "idiopathic thrombocytopenic purpura" with a family member—clear communication is crucial, but the jargon creates distance. The nuanced meaning, often lost in translation, can lead to misunderstandings with potentially serious consequences. This isn't just about semantics; it's about building trust and ensuring that everyone involved shares a common understanding.

The use of precise terminology is not inherently problematic; instead, the challenge lies in the context and the audience. Within specialized settings, the concise nature of jargon speeds up processes and enhances the accuracy of conversations. Imagine engineers discussing a "PID controller" – utilizing this jargon allows them to quickly and efficiently convey complex technical details without unnecessary elaboration. However, when this same jargon is thrown at a non-engineer, the resulting confusion undermines the purpose of communication. The key isn't to avoid jargon entirely but to exercise careful judgment regarding its appropriate use.

Mastering jargon isn't simply a matter of memorizing definitions; it's about understanding the underlying concepts. Rote learning may temporarily boost vocabulary, but true comprehension allows for flexible and appropriate application. When you truly understand the 'why' behind a term, you are better equipped to use it effectively, tailoring your language to the audience to maximize clarity and comprehension. Think of it like learning a musical instrument—memorizing scales is essential, but true musicality emerges from understanding the underlying theory and the emotional impact of the music.

This nuanced application necessitates contextual awareness. A seasoned financial analyst might readily discuss "leveraged buyouts" with colleagues. But explaining the same concept to an inexperienced investor demands a different approach, one that prioritizes clarity and avoids overwhelming them with technicalities. Effective communication isn't about showcasing knowledge; it's about sharing understanding. The ability to seamlessly shift between technical precision and accessible explanation is a key element of professional competence.

Furthermore, the evolving nature of jargon demands continuous learning. New terms, acronyms, and expressions constantly emerge within every field, reflecting advancements and shifts in understanding. Staying current with these changes is vital for professionals to maintain relevance and to effectively engage in discussions. Failure to do so can result in miscommunication, misinterpretations, and missed opportunities. Regular engagement with relevant literature, professional networks, and educational resources helps to mitigate these risks. The professional landscape is ever-shifting; mastering jargon needs to mirror this adaptability.

Consider the differences in jargon across fields. The financial world thrives on acronyms and complex financial instruments, with each possessing layers of implicit meanings. Legal discourse often involves specialized vocabulary that can quickly create bewilderment for anyone outside the legal profession. Medical language, with its dense anatomical and diagnostic terminologies, can be similarly impenetrable to the uninitiated. However, understanding this diversity is key—the same word can have vastly different meanings in various contexts. Developing awareness of this variability enhances one's ability to navigate the diverse landscape of professional communication.

Ultimately, the responsible use of jargon relies on empathy and a commitment to inclusivity. It's not about abandoning precision but about finding balance between clarity and technicality. Recognizing your audience and adapting your language to fit their level of understanding is paramount. The goal is to foster effective communication, and this involves choosing words that bridge understanding rather than build walls. To achieve this, you need to embrace adaptability and develop a keen awareness of your audience.

The consequences of misusing jargon can be far-reaching. In healthcare, misunderstandings can lead to errors in treatment, potentially jeopardizing patient outcomes. In legal contexts, misinterpretations can have serious legal repercussions, impacting decisions and judicial processes. Within business settings, imprecise communication can lead to failed negotiations, loss of contracts, and significant financial implications. By recognizing the potential impact of jargon, one can prioritize clarity and precision, ultimately mitigating these risks.

However, it's not just about avoiding jargon altogether. Some fields inherently demand a certain level of specialized language. This highlights the importance of mastering jargon within one's chosen field while also possessing the skill to translate complex ideas into simple, accessible language for audiences outside the specialized context. The ability to switch seamlessly between both levels of communication is a crucial professional asset.

Therefore, approaching jargon with awareness, respect, and adaptability is key. It's about understanding its power and limitations, and using it responsibly to ensure clear and effective communication. By recognizing the context, audience, and potential impact of jargon, professionals can use language strategically to bridge understanding and foster collaboration. The ultimate goal is clear and unambiguous communication, regardless of the audience's familiarity with specialized terminology. The intelligent use of jargon—knowing when to use it and when to translate—is a hallmark of a competent professional.

2 Medical Terminology

Understanding medical terminology can feel like deciphering a secret code, but mastering its basics opens doors to clearer communication and a deeper understanding of health and disease. It's not just about memorizing long words; it's about grasping the underlying logic and structure that makes this language work. For instance, prefixes often indicate location or direction (like "epi" meaning upon or above, as in epidermis), while suffixes denote a condition or procedure (such as "-itis" meaning inflammation, as in appendicitis). This framework facilitates learning and recall, making the seemingly overwhelming task significantly more manageable.

Learning roots, the core of many medical terms, is paramount. Consider "cardio," meaning heart, and "pulmonary," referring to the lungs. These roots form the basis for countless terms related to cardiovascular and respiratory systems, for example, "cardiomyopathy" (heart muscle disease) and "pulmonary edema" (fluid in the lungs). By understanding these core elements, you can break down unfamiliar terms into comprehensible parts, dramatically improving your comprehension and ability to confidently participate in healthcare discussions.

Medical professionals frequently use abbreviations to streamline communication, especially in fast-paced environments. While convenient for experienced practitioners, these shortcuts can be extremely confusing for the uninitiated. Common examples include "CBC" (complete blood count), "BP" (blood pressure), and "ECG" (electrocardiogram). Learning these acronyms is essential for navigating medical records, conversations, and literature. Regular exposure to medical texts and discussions is vital to internalizing the meaning and usage of these abbreviations. However, always prioritize understanding the full term before relying solely on the abbreviation. Otherwise, misinterpretations are easily made.

Disease processes often involve complex descriptions of pathophysiology, the mechanisms of disease. Comprehending the language used to explain these processes can seem daunting, yet breaking it down systematically proves helpful. Terms like "ischemia" (reduced blood flow) and "necrosis" (tissue death) are foundational concepts in understanding various ailments. Understanding the precise terminology surrounding these processes helps one comprehend not only the disease itself, but also the rationale behind treatment strategies. It illuminates the intricate connection between symptoms, diagnostic tests, and therapeutic interventions. For example, comprehending the pathophysiology of heart failure clarifies the reason for certain diagnostic tests and medications.

The field of medical treatment provides a wide array of procedures and therapies. Each has its specific terminology that needs careful consideration. Terms like "surgery," "chemotherapy," and "radiation therapy" may seem self-explanatory, but each encompasses a range of specialized techniques and procedures, with their own intricate vo-

cabulary. Learning about different surgical approaches, chemotherapy regimens, and radiation protocols requires thorough research and study, usually from reliable medical sources like textbooks and journals. The terms can appear complex, especially when dealing with highly specialized treatments such as targeted therapy or immunotherapy. However, breaking down the terms into their fundamental components—identifying roots, prefixes, and suffixes—can assist in understanding the overall therapeutic approach.
Finally, the language used in medical imaging reports often contains specific descriptions of anatomical structures and observed abnormalities. Understanding the basics of radiological terminology, for example, terms relating to location or specific types of tissue (such as "hypodense" or "hyperdense" in CT scans), significantly improves the comprehension of imaging reports. This understanding also enhances the ability to participate more actively in discussions with healthcare professionals about one's health, particularly in areas like radiology and pathology. Even basic familiarity with this language enables individuals to ask more informed questions and better understand their diagnoses and treatment plans. While complete mastery requires extensive training, developing a fundamental understanding is achievable with consistent effort and focused learning.

2.1 Anatomy Basics

Understanding the human body begins with its fundamental building blocks: cells, tissues, organs, and organ systems. These structures work together in a complex and coordinated manner, performing specialized functions crucial for maintaining life. Mastering the terminology associated with these structures is fundamental to comprehending medical discussions, whether you're a healthcare professional or simply aiming to become a more informed patient. For example, knowing the difference between "anterior" and "posterior" is key, as these terms refer to the front and back of the body, respectively, a fundamental directional term widely used in anatomical descriptions. Similarly, terms like "superior" and "inferior" indicating above and below, respectively, are essential for clear communication about anatomical locations.

The body is organized hierarchically. Cells, the basic units of life, combine to form tissues. Tissues group together to create organs, and organs work together to form organ systems. Each level exhibits its own unique features and functions. For instance, epithelial tissue covers body surfaces and forms glands; connective tissue supports and connects different parts of the body; muscular tissue enables movement; and nervous tissue transmits electrical signals. Understanding these tissue types is crucial for recognizing the basic building blocks of organs. Consider, for example, the heart: It's composed of cardiac muscle tissue, which allows it to pump blood. The heart is an organ, but it's part of the cardiovascular system – a larger functional unit coordinating blood circulation throughout the body.

Medical professionals frequently utilize prefixes and suffixes to construct complex terms. These elements help to break down lengthy, seemingly intimidating medical terms into smaller, more manageable parts. Take, for example, the word "cardiomyopathy." "Cardio" refers to the heart; "myo" refers to muscle; and "-pathy" signifies disease. Therefore, cardiomyopathy translates to "heart muscle disease." Learning common prefixes and suffixes will greatly improve your ability to decipher medical jargon. This technique of understanding root words and their prefixes/suffixes allows the quick understanding of numerous terms. Understanding "gastr-" (stomach) and "-itis" (inflammation) will allow you to understand that "gastritis" refers to stomach inflammation; similarly, combining "hepat-" (liver) with "-itis" will easily reveal the meaning of "hepatitis". Mastering these fundamental elements is the cornerstone of understanding medical terminology.

Anatomical planes of reference are another crucial aspect. These planes—sagittal, frontal (coronal), and transverse (axial)—are used to describe the location of structures within the body. The sagittal plane divides the body into left and right halves, the frontal plane divides the body into front and back, and the transverse plane divides the body into upper and lower sections. These planes of section are used in imaging techniques such as MRI and CT scans to visualize internal organs and structures, so understanding the location of a lesion described as being in a certain plane is crucial for interpretation. Precise communication about the location of pathologies needs these common references; without them, the identification of lesions could become far more challenging.

Finally, regional anatomy focuses on specific regions of the body, like the head, neck, thorax, abdomen, and limbs. Each region has its unique structures and terminology. For example, knowing the difference between the brachial (arm) and antebrachial (forearm) regions is essential for accurate communication about injuries or conditions affecting those areas. Thoracic anatomy encompasses structures within the chest cavity such as the heart, lungs, and great vessels. Abdominal anatomy details organs within the abdomen, like the liver, stomach, intestines, and kidneys. While the study of anatomy can initially seem daunting, understanding the basic principles of anatomical organization—from the cellular to the systemic level—forms a vital foundation for comprehending the intricacies of the human body and interpreting medical jargon more effectively. The systematic approach to learning, breaking down complex terms, and understanding regional anatomy provides a powerful framework for medical terminology mastery.

2.2 Disease Processes

Understanding disease processes requires grasping specific terminology. Think of it like learning a new language, but instead of verbs and nouns, we have prefixes, suffixes, and root words that describe the body's malfunctioning. For instance, "itis" always signals inflammation; appendicitis, therefore, points directly to inflammation of the appendix. This knowledge dramatically accelerates comprehension of medical reports and discussions.

Many diseases follow predictable patterns. Acute illnesses, like influenza, strike suddenly and often resolve relatively quickly. Chronic conditions, in contrast, such as diabetes or hypertension, persist over extended periods. Recognizing this distinction is crucial; treatment strategies differ drastically between acute and chronic illnesses. A short course of antiviral medication might suffice for influenza, while diabetes management necessitates lifelong adjustments in diet and possibly medication. This categorization isn't rigid, though; some conditions transition from acute to chronic states.

Furthermore, consider the etiology of disease – the study of its causes. Infectious diseases stem from pathogenic microorganisms, like bacteria or viruses. Genetic diseases arise from inherited defects in an individual's DNA. Environmental factors, such as exposure to toxins, also play a substantial role. Understanding the etiology helps us predict the disease's progression and guide prevention efforts. For example, understanding the viral nature of influenza facilitates the development of vaccines and antiviral treatments. Similarly, knowledge of genetic predispositions allows for early screening and preventative measures for certain diseases.

The pathogenesis – the process of disease development – is equally important. It outlines the cellular and molecular events that lead to observable symptoms. Take atherosclerosis, the buildup of plaque in arteries. The pathogenesis involves complex interactions between cholesterol, inflammation, and the endothelium, the lining of blood vessels. Understanding this progression allows clinicians to target specific steps in the process with medication, slowing or halting the disease's advance. In simpler terms, instead of merely treating symptoms, understanding pathogenesis helps target the underlying cause of the illness.

Clinical manifestations, or the outward signs and symptoms, help diagnose diseases. These include physical findings like fever, rash, or altered heart sounds; and lab results such as elevated white blood cell counts or abnormal enzyme levels. Correlating clinical manifestations with the disease's pathogenesis paints a comprehensive picture. For example, a patient presenting with chest pain, shortness of breath, and elevated cardiac enzymes strongly suggests a myocardial infarction (heart attack). Recognizing these connections is fundamental to correct diagnosis and timely intervention.

The progression of a disease isn't always straightforward. Some conditions follow predictable patterns, while others exhibit variability. Remission, a period where symptoms subside, is common in many diseases, such as cancer. Conversely, exacerbations, periods of increased severity, can occur, often requiring adjusted treatment. It's essential to acknowledge that each individual responds differently to disease, emphasizing the importance of personalized approaches to management.

Finally, remember the significance of prognosis. This refers to the predicted course and outcome of a disease. Prognosis is influenced by various factors, including the disease's severity, the patient's overall health, and the response to treatment. While prognosis offers valuable insights, it's crucial to avoid fatalism. Advances in medical treatment constantly refine our understanding and improve outcomes. A detailed prognosis provides a framework for making informed decisions about treatment options and end-of-life care where appropriate. The focus should always remain on managing the condition and enhancing the patient's quality of life, even in the face of a challenging prognosis.

2.3 Treatment Options

Surgical procedures encompass a vast array of techniques, each with its own specialized vocabulary. From minimally invasive laparoscopic surgeries, employing terms like "trocar insertion" and "pneumoperitoneum," to complex open-heart procedures utilizing phrases like "cardiopulmonary bypass" and "aortic valve replacement," understanding the terminology is crucial for patient comprehension and informed consent. The descriptions often involve intricate details of the surgical approach, the instruments used, and the specific anatomical structures involved. For example, a description of a coronary artery bypass graft might include references to internal mammary arteries, saphenous veins, and anastomosis. This level of detail, while essential for medical professionals, can be daunting for patients. Therefore, clear and concise explanations tailored to the patient's understanding are critical.

Understanding the nuances of pharmaceutical terminology is equally important. This isn't simply about knowing the generic and brand names of drugs. It's about grasping the concepts of drug administration routes—oral, intravenous, subcutaneous—and understanding the meaning of terms like "pharmacokinetics" (the body's effect on the drug) and "pharmacodynamics" (the drug's effect on the body). Moreover, knowing the different types of drug interactions, like synergistic or antagonistic effects, is vital for effective treatment. One must also understand the terminology around dosage forms—tablets, capsules, solutions, suspensions—and how those forms impact drug absorption and efficacy. This is essential for patients to adhere to their prescribed medication regimens and to communicate effectively with their healthcare providers about any side effects or concerns.

Radiation therapy, another crucial treatment modality, presents its own linguistic challenges. Understanding the difference between external beam radiation therapy and brachytherapy (internal radiation) is fundamental. Beyond these distinctions, patients need to be familiar with terms like "radiation dose," "fractionation," and "target volume," all of which are central to the treatment planning process. Moreover, the potential side effects, often described using sophisticated medical terminology, need to be explained clearly to patients. The potential for fatigue, nausea, skin reactions, and other complications must be explained in plain language to manage patient expectations and support their coping mechanisms. Open communication and plain language are essential to ensure a patient's understanding and cooperation throughout the treatment.

Beyond surgery, pharmaceuticals, and radiation, there's a growing emphasis on integrative and alternative medicine approaches. These methods frequently employ their own unique terminology, requiring an additional layer of understanding. Terms such as "acupuncture meridians," "herbal remedies," "homeopathic dilutions," and "mindfulness techniques" may be unfamiliar to those outside of these fields. The efficacy and safety of these alternative treatments are often debated, further highlighting the necessity of clear communication between patients and practitioners to prevent misunderstandings and ensure the best possible treatment outcome. This emphasizes the necessity of medical professionals to adapt their vocabulary to ensure effective communication with patients.

Finally, understanding the language of diagnostics is critical in the treatment planning process. This includes understanding the various imaging modalities, their terminology, and their purpose. From X-rays and CT scans to MRI and PET scans, each technique provides different views of the body's internal structures, using unique terminology that patients often struggle to grasp. The interpretation of these images—a critical step in diagnosis and treatment planning—often utilizes terms that describe findings, like “lesion,” “mass,” “nodule,” or “metastasis.” It's important for patients to understand these terms and the implications for their treatment so they can actively participate in their healthcare. Effectively communicating diagnostic findings requires careful consideration of the patient's understanding and a willingness to provide clear and concise explanations. Building trust and fostering open communication are essential for successful medical treatment.

3 Legal Language

Understanding legal language is crucial, not just for lawyers, but for anyone interacting with the legal system. A basic grasp of common terms can prevent misunderstandings and empower you to navigate legal documents and situations with greater confidence. This is especially true given the inherent complexity and formality embedded within legal jargon.

Consider the simple phrase "habeas corpus." While seemingly arcane, it represents a fundamental right—the right to challenge unlawful imprisonment. Understanding this term allows you to recognize situations where this right might be violated and to know how to seek appropriate legal recourse. Similarly, understanding the difference between "felony" and "misdemeanor" is vital for assessing the seriousness of a crime and its potential consequences. These are not abstract legal concepts but have significant real-world implications.

Contract law, in particular, utilizes a unique vocabulary. Terms such as "consideration," "breach of contract," and "force majeure" are frequently encountered. "Consideration," for instance, refers to something of value exchanged between parties to a contract, making the agreement legally binding. Without understanding this basic principle, you might inadvertently enter into a non-binding contract, leaving you without legal recourse. Similarly, "breach of contract" describes a failure to fulfill the obligations outlined in the contract, potentially leading to legal action. Recognizing these terms will be critical in preventing costly legal troubles. Moreover, familiarity with the concept of "force majeure"—an unforeseen event beyond one's control, such as a natural disaster—is crucial when navigating complex commercial agreements, potentially allowing for the renegotiation of contractual obligations in extraordinary circumstances.

Legal research demands its own specialized language. Knowing how to effectively use legal databases and understand citation formats (like Bluebook or ALWD) is essential for locating relevant case law and statutes. The ability to decipher these legal citations is not simply a technical skill, but it's a necessary tool for anyone looking to gain a solid understanding of legal precedent or the reasoning behind particular judicial rulings. Comprehending the difference between a "statute" and a "case" – one being a law passed by a legislature and the other being a judicial decision interpreting such a law – is fundamental to legal research. This distinction is often not immediately apparent to those unfamiliar with the legal field, yet it is crucial for effective legal analysis.

Navigating criminal justice terms is particularly important for anyone who might find themselves involved in the justice system, whether as a victim, a witness, or even a defendant. Understanding terms like "arraignment," "plea bargain," and "habeas corpus" (mentioned earlier) is essential for comprehending the procedures involved in a criminal case. For example, "arraignment" is the formal reading of criminal charges, while a "plea bargain" involves a defendant agreeing to plead guilty in exchange for a reduced sentence. These terms and the processes they represent are fundamental to the way the system works and understanding them is crucial in participating in the legal system effectively. Even a basic understanding of these terms can improve one's understanding of the news and better equip individuals to understand their rights if involved in the legal process.

Civil law encompasses a broad range of legal disputes, from contract breaches to personal injury claims. Terms like "negligence," "liability," and "damages" are essential for understanding civil lawsuits. "Negligence," for example, is the failure to exercise the care that a reasonably prudent person would exercise in a similar situation; its presence or absence is crucial in determining liability in many personal injury cases. Likewise, "damages" represent the monetary compensation awarded to a party who has suffered a loss or injury due to another party's actions. Grasping these concepts is important, not just for lawyers, but for anyone who might be involved in a civil dispute.

In conclusion, while legal language can appear daunting, developing even a rudimentary understanding of key terms offers significant benefits. This knowledge enhances your ability to participate actively in legal processes, understand legal documents, and advocate effectively for your rights. Mastering this specialized vocabulary isn't about becoming a lawyer, but rather, about equipping yourself with the tools to navigate a world where legal considerations are inevitably present. Becoming more familiar with legal language makes you a more informed and empowered individual, allowing you to engage with legal matters confidently and understand the implications they may have on your life.

3.1 Courtroom Jargon

The hushed reverence of a courtroom is palpable; a tension hangs in the air, thick with unspoken expectations. Every word, every gesture, holds weight. Understanding the language—the jargon—is crucial for anyone navigating this environment, whether as a participant or an observer. This chapter aims to unravel some of this intricate legal lexicon, offering a beginner's guide to courtroom terminology.

"Objection, hearsay!" This phrase, a common courtroom staple, signifies a challenge to the admissibility of evidence. Hearsay is generally defined as secondhand information, something someone told a witness rather than the witness's direct observation. Understanding this objection – and countless others – is essential for comprehending the flow of a trial. The judge's ruling on such an objection dictates whether or not the information can be considered by the jury. A successful objection could completely alter the course of the proceedings. Therefore, the accurate and timely use of such objections is a crucial aspect of courtroom procedure. The legal system, in essence, functions on the precise usage and understanding of these terms.

Beyond objections, consider the concept of voir dire. This is the process of jury selection, where attorneys question potential jurors to assess their biases and suitability. It's a crucial stage, as a biased jury can dramatically affect the outcome of a case. Attorneys carefully pick jurors, seeking those who appear impartial and will engage in fair deliberation. Questions posed during voir dire can range from personal beliefs on justice to specific views on the type of case being presented. This process demonstrates the careful consideration that goes into the foundational aspects of a trial. The impact of carefully selected jurors or inadvertently biased ones can affect a case significantly. This is a powerful example of why mastering courtroom jargon is paramount for success within the legal system.

Then there's the matter of direct examination and cross-examination. Direct examination is the initial questioning of a witness by the attorney who called them. The attorney aims to elicit favorable testimony, presenting the witness's version of events. Cross-examination, however, follows, wherein the opposing attorney attempts to discredit the witness's testimony and highlight inconsistencies. Both are critical stages, as the presentation of evidence depends greatly on this dynamic. Each interaction shapes the narrative of the trial, revealing layers of truth (or manufactured truths). The distinction between these two processes highlights the adversarial nature of legal proceedings. Effective use of these distinct questioning styles, along with understanding their differences, is crucial for winning your case.

We also need to consider the significance of depositions. These are pre-trial sworn statements taken from witnesses. Their importance lies in their ability to gather information and lock down witness accounts before the trial itself. Attorneys utilize depositions to prepare for trial, to expose potential inconsistencies or weaknesses in the opposing side's case. Often, inconsistencies found in depositions can be used effectively during cross-examination. Therefore, taking notes accurately and keeping detailed records is essential. A meticulous attorney anticipates many questions an opposing counsel may ask. This proactive strategy helps strengthen the entire legal team's position within the court. In a word, the preparation found within this step of a case is integral to the

courtroom proceeding.
Finally, let's not overlook the significance of summation, or closing arguments. This is the final opportunity for each side to present their case, summarizing evidence and arguing for a verdict in their favor. Effective summation involves expertly weaving together the threads of the trial, highlighting key evidence and persuading the jury to accept their version of the facts. This phase requires both legal acumen and persuasive communication skills. It requires the skillful integration of collected evidence, well-structured arguments and emotionally persuasive delivery. The impact of a powerful summation cannot be overstated. The ability to present a compelling argument is essential in influencing the jury. The successful attorney masters this aspect of trial proceedings and knows this is the last chance to impress upon the judge and jury the truth of their case. The impact of a persuasive summation should not be underestimated.

3.2 Contract Law Terms

Consider the significance of "offer" and "acceptance" in forming a legally binding contract. These aren't mere suggestions; they represent the cornerstone of agreement. An offer must be clear, definite, and communicate a willingness to enter into a contract. Ambiguity, vague language, or statements expressing mere intent are not considered valid offers. Think of it like this: if I say, "I might sell you my car," that isn't an offer. However, "I offer to sell you my car for $10,000" is a clear and definite offer, ready for acceptance.
Acceptance, similarly, requires unequivocal agreement to the terms of

the offer. A counter-offer, modifying any aspect of the original offer, effectively rejects it and creates a new offer. Imagine negotiating a salary: You receive an offer of $60,000. Responding with, "I'll accept if you raise it to $65,000," constitutes a counter-offer, nullifying the original offer. Silence generally doesn't imply acceptance, unless prior dealings between the parties established it as such.

The concept of "consideration" is crucial. It's the mutual exchange of something of value, forming the backbone of a contract's enforceability. This could be money, goods, services, or even a promise to do or refrain from doing something. A mere gratuitous promise, lacking consideration, is usually unenforceable. For example, promising to give a friend a gift is not a binding contract because there's no reciprocal obligation. The consideration must be sufficient, not necessarily adequate, meaning it holds some legal value, however small.

"Capacity" refers to the legal ability of a party to enter into a contract. Minors, individuals deemed mentally incapacitated, or those under duress lack the capacity to form a valid contract. Their contracts are often voidable, meaning they can be rescinded. Imagine a minor signing a contract for a large loan – that contract could be challenged and potentially voided. Understanding capacity is vital, particularly when dealing with vulnerable individuals.

Understanding the principle of "legality" is paramount. Contracts that involve illegal activities or violate public policy are void and unenforceable. A contract to commit a crime, for instance, is clearly void. This principle underscores the importance of ensuring that the subject matter of any contract falls within the boundaries of the law. Ignoring legality can lead to severe consequences.

The interpretation of contract terms, particularly ambiguous ones, is guided by various rules of construction. Courts often favor interpretations that avoid absurdity or injustice. This principle ensures fairness and aims to reflect the parties' likely intentions. The "parol evidence rule," generally barring extrinsic evidence contradicting a written contract's terms, reinforces the importance of clear, written agreements. This rule helps to provide clarity and prevent disputes arising from contradictory evidence.

Finally, remember that even a seemingly flawless contract can be affected by unforeseen events. The "doctrine of frustration" recognizes that contracts can become impossible to perform due to events beyond the parties' control, leading to discharge of the contract. Imagine a venue booking cancelled due to a natural disaster – the contract might be frustrated, releasing both parties from their obligations. Thorough contract drafting can mitigate such risks but cannot eliminate them entirely. Anticipating potential disruptions and including carefully worded clauses can help protect parties' interests. It is vital to seek legal counsel when drafting or reviewing contracts of any significant value or complexity to ensure they adequately reflect your needs and are legally sound. Failing to do so can lead to costly and time-consuming disputes down the line, highlighting the importance of understanding the specific legal terminology involved. Ignoring these aspects can have severe financial and legal repercussions. Professional legal advice is highly recommended to navigate this complex area of the law.

3.3 Criminal Justice Terms

Understanding criminal justice terminology is crucial for anyone interacting with the legal system, whether as a professional or a concerned citizen. Terms like "arraignment," "plea bargain," and "habeas corpus" are frequently encountered, yet their precise meanings often remain elusive to the uninitiated. This chapter aims to clarify some of these core concepts, providing a foundation for navigating the complexities of criminal proceedings.

The process begins with an arrest. This doesn't automatically mean a conviction. Following arrest, the accused is typically brought before a judge for an arraignment. During this formal hearing, charges are read, rights are explained (often including the right to remain silent and the right to legal counsel), and bail may be set. Understanding the difference between bail and bond is vital; bail is the money or property guaranteeing your appearance in court, while a bond is issued by a surety company. Misunderstanding these terms can lead to unnecessary complications and potentially significant financial burdens.

Next, consider the concept of a plea bargain. This is a negotiation between the prosecution and the defense, where the accused agrees to plead guilty to a lesser charge in exchange for a reduced sentence or other concessions. These negotiations, often conducted behind closed doors, can drastically impact the outcome of a case. The complexities involved highlight the need for skilled legal representation, capable of weighing the risks and benefits of such agreements. A successful plea bargain can mean avoiding a lengthy and expensive trial, potentially saving time and resources for both the defendant and the judicial system. However, it also means surrendering certain rights, a trade-off demanding careful consideration.

Beyond arraignment and plea bargains, the legal system utilizes a plethora of specific terms. For instance, "habeas corpus" is a legal action used to challenge the legality of a person's detention or imprisonment. This fundamental legal right protects individuals from unlawful confinement, ensuring that their imprisonment is justified by legal process. Similarly, understanding the nuances of "ex post facto" laws, which criminalize actions committed before the law was enacted, is crucial for appreciating the principles of due process. These protections are fundamental cornerstones of a fair legal system, preventing arbitrary punishment.

Evidence is another key concept, with distinctions between direct and circumstantial evidence. Direct evidence directly proves a fact, such as eyewitness testimony. Circumstantial evidence, on the other hand, implies a fact; for example, finding a suspect's fingerprints at a crime scene. The weight given to each type of evidence can vary significantly depending on the specifics of the case and the judge's interpretation. A thorough understanding of these distinctions is vital for interpreting trial proceedings accurately. Judges and juries carefully weigh this evidence to make well-informed decisions. The ability to differentiate between various forms of evidence and understand their relative strengths and weaknesses is fundamental to effective legal analysis.

Finally, sentencing itself involves a range of terms. Sentences may be concurrent (served simultaneously) or consecutive (served one after another). They can range from probation (supervised release) to incarceration in various levels of security. These sentences reflect the severity of the crime and the judge's assessment of the defendant's culpability and potential for rehabilitation. Mandatory minimum sentences, where a specific minimum prison term is required by law, are also relevant here. The specifics of sentencing can be complex, influenced by a variety of factors including criminal history, mitigating and aggravating circumstances, and the nature of the offense. Understanding these complexities empowers individuals to engage more effectively with the criminal justice system and to follow legal proceedings with a higher degree of comprehension. Proper legal counsel is usually essential for navigating the intricacies of sentencing to achieve the best possible outcomes.

3.4 Civil Law Terms

Plaintiffs initiate civil lawsuits, seeking remedies for alleged wrongs. Understanding the terminology is crucial, as it forms the foundation of legal arguments and court proceedings. For instance, a "complaint" formally outlines the plaintiff's claims, while an "answer" represents the defendant's response. These initial pleadings set the stage for the legal battle to come, establishing the core issues and defenses involved. The process, while often complex, hinges on a clear understanding of these fundamental terms.

Jurisdiction, a term frequently encountered, refers to the court's authority to hear a specific case. Federal courts have jurisdiction over cases involving federal law, while state courts address state law matters. Concurrent jurisdiction exists when both federal and state courts can hear a case. This complexity underscores the importance of understanding jurisdictional boundaries for choosing the appropriate venue for a lawsuit. Navigating the intricacies of jurisdiction is a key skill for legal professionals and informed citizens alike.

Evidence plays a pivotal role in civil litigation, with its admissibility governed by strict rules. Relevant evidence, tending to prove or disprove a fact in question, is generally admissible. However, hearsay, or statements made outside of court, is typically inadmissible unless it falls under a recognized exception. This complex interplay between admissibility and relevance can significantly impact a case's outcome, highlighting the necessity for a firm grasp of evidentiary rules. Proper understanding of what is considered admissible evidence is crucial in shaping the course of any civil lawsuit.

Discovery, a crucial pre-trial phase, involves the exchange of information between parties. This process often uses interrogatories, written questions requiring written answers, and depositions, sworn oral testimonies given under oath. Requests for production of documents compel the disclosure of relevant materials. This robust information exchange aims to promote fairness and prevent trial by ambush, ensuring that both sides have access to pertinent information before the trial begins. This phase of investigation in advance, enables better preparation and ultimately leads to a more informed, just outcome.

Damages, the financial compensation awarded to a prevailing plaintiff, can be compensatory, designed to cover actual losses, or punitive, intended to punish the defendant for egregious conduct. Compensatory damages may include medical expenses, lost wages, and pain and suffering. Punitive damages, on the other hand, aim to deter similar future conduct and are awarded only in cases of particularly egregious misconduct. The determination of appropriate damages often requires a careful assessment of both the plaintiff's losses and the defendant's actions. The calculation of damages is a critical aspect of many civil cases.

Settlement negotiations often occur before trial, aiming to resolve disputes without the expense and uncertainty of litigation. Parties might engage in mediation, a neutral third-party assists in facilitating a compromise. Arbitration, a more formal process, involves a neutral party who hears evidence and renders a binding decision. Settlement negotiations offer an alternative dispute resolution (ADR) approach that often proves efficient and cost-effective. Choosing between mediation and arbitration and understanding the specific details of each method will assist a more efficient approach to problem solving.

Finally, appeals represent a potential next step after an adverse judgment. An appellate court reviews the lower court's decision for errors of law. The appellate process offers a chance to challenge the lower court's ruling, providing a crucial safeguard in the judicial system. If a court determines an error occurred in the judgment, a trial may need to be repeated. These complex procedures highlight the multi-layered nature of the civil justice system, offering both protection and opportunity for appeal. The appellate process can be time-consuming and complex, requiring specific legal knowledge and strategic planning. An informed understanding of this process is of extreme importance.

3.5 Legal Research

Legal research can seem daunting, especially for those unfamiliar with the intricacies of legal databases and terminology. It's a skill honed over time, but understanding the basics significantly improves your ability to find relevant information efficiently. The key is to develop a strategic approach, breaking down the process into manageable steps.

Begin with a clear understanding of your research question. Vague queries yield vague results. Precisely define the issue you're investigating; formulating your research question clearly, you'll be better able to target keywords and search terms that will result in a more effective and efficient search. This initial step is crucial because it guides the entire research process. A poorly defined question leads to wasted time and potentially flawed conclusions.

Once your question is framed, identifying relevant keywords is critical. Think about the key terms and concepts that define your research area. Consider synonyms, related terms, and broader concepts. This comprehensive approach maximizes your chances of finding relevant information in legal databases which can often contain very specific information, requiring you to look for the specific term or even the specific legal form. Legal databases are your primary tool, offering comprehensive access to case law, statutes, regulations, and scholarly articles. Westlaw, LexisNexis, and Bloomberg Law are industry giants, each with unique features and search capabilities. Familiarize yourself with their interfaces and advanced search functions.

Knowing how to effectively utilize Boolean operators – AND, OR, NOT – is essential. These operators allow you to refine your searches, narrowing or broadening your results to identify the information you need. For instance, combining "contract" AND "breach" AND "damages" significantly narrows your results compared to searching for those terms individually. Mastering this technique will significantly improve the precision and efficiency of your research process. It's a basic step, but many overlook its power and end up with a huge number of useless results that they have to sift through.

Don't overlook secondary sources. While primary sources (case law, statutes) are central, legal textbooks, scholarly articles, and legal encyclopedias provide valuable context and analysis. These sources offer an interpretation and understanding of the primary sources, often in a form which might prove to be easier to use and to understand the content. These secondary sources offer crucial background information and provide differing perspectives, enriching your understanding of the legal issues at hand.

Remember to properly cite your sources. This is not merely an academic formality; it's crucial for maintaining accuracy and giving credit to original authors. Different legal citation styles exist (e.g., Bluebook, ALWD), and adhering to the appropriate style demonstrates your commitment to scholarly integrity and professional standards. This includes the accurate reproduction of every single word, making sure that there aren't any mistakes that might influence the content. A missed citation can damage your credibility, a detail that is as important as it might seem.

Finally, continuously evaluate your research process. What strategies worked best? What challenges did you face? Refining your approach based on experience is key to becoming an efficient legal researcher.

Keep detailed records of your search terms, databases, and sources; this practice not only aids in replication but also highlights areas for improvement in your workflow. This will help you not only to be faster but also to gain an awareness of the entire process, making you more efficient and self-aware as a legal researcher. The more you search, the more you will adapt your research style, so be sure to keep your mind open and keep experimenting.

4 Financial Jargon

Understanding financial jargon is crucial for navigating the modern world. Whether you're planning for retirement, investing in the stock market, or simply trying to decipher a bank statement, a grasp of these terms is essential for informed decision-making. Ignoring financial jargon leaves you vulnerable to misinformation and potentially costly mistakes. It's like trying to assemble furniture without instructions; you might manage, but it will likely be inefficient and potentially frustrating.

Let's start with investments. You'll frequently encounter terms like "stocks," "bonds," and "mutual funds." Stocks represent ownership in a company, their value fluctuating with the company's performance. Bonds, on the other hand, are loans you make to a company or government, earning interest over time. Mutual funds pool money from multiple investors to invest in a diversified portfolio of stocks, bonds, or other assets, spreading risk and offering professional management – a significant advantage for less experienced investors. Understanding these distinctions is fundamental to making sound investment choices. Don't simply rely on others' advice; learn the basics yourself.

Moving on to banking, you'll need to familiarize yourself with concepts like "interest rates," "APR," and "compound interest." Interest rates determine how much you earn on savings or pay on loans. APR, or Annual Percentage Rate, represents the annual cost of borrowing, encompassing interest and other fees. Compound interest, often considered the eighth wonder of the world, involves earning interest not only on your principal but also on accumulated interest, resulting in exponential growth over time. Mastering these concepts will allow you to make informed decisions about loans, mortgages, and savings accounts, potentially saving you thousands in the long run. Don't be afraid to ask your bank or financial advisor to explain these concepts clearly, and don't settle for vague answers.

Understanding financial statements is another vital skill. Learning to interpret balance sheets, income statements, and cash flow statements is like learning to read a map; it will allow you to navigate the financial landscape with confidence. A balance sheet provides a snapshot of a company's assets, liabilities, and equity at a specific point in time. The income statement shows a company's revenues and expenses over a period, revealing profitability. Finally, the cash flow statement tracks the movement of cash into and out of a company. These documents provide crucial insights into a company's financial health, crucial for making smart investment decisions and understanding economic reports.

Furthermore, delving into terms like "diversification," "risk tolerance," and "asset allocation" is crucial for building a strong financial foundation. Diversification involves spreading investments across various asset classes to mitigate risk. Risk tolerance reflects your comfort level with potential investment losses. Asset allocation determines how your investments are distributed across different asset classes, like stocks, bonds, and real estate. These considerations are paramount in building a portfolio suited to your individual circumstances and risk profile. Never invest based purely on someone else's recommendations; thorough research and informed decisions are key.

Finally, let's not overlook the importance of understanding market indices like the Dow Jones Industrial Average and the S&P 500. These indices track the performance of a group of selected stocks, offering a broader view of the market. Keeping up with these metrics allows you to monitor the overall health of the market and make informed decisions about your investment strategy. Watching market fluctuations can seem daunting at first; however, gradually learn to interpret them. The news is full of financial jargon, and without understanding the basics, you're only half-informed. Understanding these market indicators is crucial to staying informed and making sound investment choices in the long run. The financial world offers numerous opportunities for growth and security, but only with knowledge and diligent research can you truly capitalize on these benefits. Investing wisely requires thorough understanding, not just blind faith or speculation.

4.1 Investing Terms

Understanding the financial world often feels like deciphering a secret code. Terms like "bull market" and "hedge fund" are thrown around casually, leaving the uninitiated feeling lost and confused. This chapter aims to demystify some of the most common investing terms, providing you with the foundational knowledge needed to navigate the world of finance with confidence. It's not about becoming a Wall Street wizard overnight; it's about equipping you with the vocabulary to understand what you're reading and hearing.

Let's start with the basics. A "stock," for instance, represents ownership in a company. When you buy a stock, you become a shareholder, entitled to a portion of the company's profits and voting rights. Conversely, a "bond" is essentially a loan you make to a company or government. They pay you interest over a set period, and then return your principal at maturity. Understanding this fundamental difference is crucial to making informed investment decisions. Your risk tolerance plays a significant role in choosing between stocks and bonds. Stocks, inherently riskier, offer potential for greater rewards. Bonds, providing stability, are usually safer but with lower returns.

Diversification is a key concept often overlooked by beginners. It's the practice of spreading your investments across different asset classes, like stocks, bonds, and real estate. This reduces your overall risk. Imagine putting all your eggs in one basket—risky, right? Diversification is your insurance policy against market fluctuations. Don't put all your money into one stock, expecting huge returns. Instead, distribute your investments across different sectors and markets, reducing dependence on a single company's performance. A balanced portfolio is essential for long-term growth.

Moving on to more advanced terms, "mutual funds" are investment vehicles that pool money from multiple investors to buy a diversified portfolio of securities. This allows you to benefit from professional management and diversification without having to make individual stock picks. Similarly, "exchange-traded funds" (ETFs) are similar to mutual funds, but they trade on stock exchanges like individual stocks, offering greater flexibility. Both provide a way to gain exposure to a market segment without the extensive research needed to select individual assets. Understanding these instruments broadens your investment options considerably.

Now, let's address some common market indicators. A "bull market" is characterized by rising prices and investor optimism. Conversely, a "bear market" is defined by falling prices and widespread pessimism. These terms reflect the overall sentiment in the market. Knowing which market you're operating in is important to adjust your investment strategy. A bull market might seem perfect for aggressive investing, while a bear market calls for a more cautious approach. Timing the market is impossible. Instead, focus on building a strong foundation and a balanced portfolio, regardless of current market trends.

"Capital gains" refer to profits earned from selling an asset, such as a stock or bond, for more than you paid for it. These gains are typically taxable. Conversely, "dividends" are payments made by companies to their shareholders, usually from profits. Both capital gains and dividends contribute to your investment returns. Remember to plan for taxes on these returns, and factor tax implications into your overall strategy. The tax laws in your jurisdiction may influence the asset allocation strategy.

Finally, let's touch upon the concept of "risk tolerance." This refers to your ability and willingness to accept potential losses in pursuit of higher returns. Different investors have different levels of risk tolerance. Some might be comfortable taking on significant risk for the chance of high rewards, while others prefer a more conservative approach. Knowing your own risk tolerance is crucial in choosing suitable investments. You need to choose what aligns with your financial situation, future goals, and personality. Avoid investments that make you anxious or uncomfortable.

Understanding these fundamental investing terms is just the first step on your journey to financial literacy. Further exploration into more specialized areas will deepen your understanding and allow you to make more informed decisions. Remember, this knowledge is a tool to empower you; responsible investment requires constant learning and careful consideration of your unique circumstances. Don't be intimidated by the jargon; use it as a means to your financial goals.

4.2 Banking Concepts

Understanding banking concepts can seem daunting, especially when confronted with unfamiliar terms. It's a field brimming with specific language, but mastering the basics is surprisingly accessible. Think of it like learning a new language; start with the common phrases, build your vocabulary gradually, and before you know it, you'll be navigating financial discussions with ease.

One of the most fundamental concepts is understanding different account types. Checking accounts offer easy access to funds, often through debit cards and checks, making them ideal for everyday transactions. Savings accounts, on the other hand, are designed for accumulating funds, typically offering slightly higher interest rates but with limitations on withdrawals. Money market accounts often combine features of both, offering higher interest rates than basic savings accounts with check-writing privileges, though sometimes with minimum balance requirements. Knowing the distinctions between these account types is crucial for effective money management.

Next, let's explore the mechanics of loans. Loans are essentially borrowed funds that require repayment, typically with interest. The interest rate, a crucial aspect of any loan, is the cost of borrowing. Lower interest rates mean lower borrowing costs, while higher rates increase the overall cost. Understanding APR (Annual Percentage Rate), which includes fees and other charges, provides a comprehensive picture of the true cost of borrowing. Different loan types exist for various purposes – mortgages for houses, auto loans for vehicles, personal loans for various needs – each with its own terms and conditions.

Credit cards, while seemingly straightforward, are intricate financial instruments. They offer short-term borrowing, letting you make purchases now and pay later. However, high interest rates and potential fees make responsible management vital. Your credit score, a crucial factor in obtaining credit, reflects your history of borrowing and repayment. A higher score usually results in better interest rates and credit limits. Understanding your credit report, and working to maintain a healthy score, is essential for accessing affordable credit in the future. Furthermore, understanding your credit utilization rate, which measures how much of your available credit you are currently using, is key to maintaining a positive credit score. Keeping your utilization rate low signals responsible credit management to lenders.

Beyond individual accounts and loans, understanding financial institutions themselves is crucial. Commercial banks offer a wide range of services to individuals and businesses, including checking and savings accounts, loans, and investment products. Credit unions, often member-owned and not-for-profit, may offer similar services but often with lower fees and more favorable interest rates for their members. Investment banks focus on providing financial services to corporations and governments, often involved in complex transactions like mergers and acquisitions. These institutions work together to create a complex financial ecosystem.

Finally, navigating the complexities of banking also involves grasping regulatory bodies. These bodies, like the Federal Reserve in the United States or similar organizations in other countries, play a vital role in regulating banks and overseeing the stability of the financial system. Understanding their function is essential for maintaining confidence in the financial system. They create and enforce rules designed to protect consumers and maintain a healthy financial environment. Staying informed about these regulations and changes within the banking landscape is crucial for making educated financial decisions and protecting your interests.

5 Technical Terminology

Understanding software development often requires navigating a sea of acronyms and technical terms. Consider the difference between "front-end" and "back-end" development; the former deals with the user interface, the part you directly interact with, while the latter manages the server-side logic and databases – the unseen engine powering the application. Grasping this distinction is crucial for anyone involved in software projects, whether as a client, manager, or even a casual observer. Failing to understand these basic distinctions could lead to miscommunication and ultimately project failure. Mastering this terminology empowers you to participate effectively in discussions, understand project specifications, and contribute meaningfully to the development process. This is not merely about memorizing definitions; it's about understanding the functional roles each component plays within the larger system. The world of computer hardware is equally replete with specialized vocabulary. Terms like "CPU," "RAM," "GPU," and "SSD" are not just jargon; they represent fundamental building blocks of any computer system. The CPU, or central processing unit, is the brain; RAM, or random-access memory, acts as short-term storage; the GPU, or graphics processing unit, handles visual processing; and the SSD, or solid-state drive, is a type of high-speed storage. Understanding the interplay of these components is vital for troubleshooting computer issues, choosing appropriate hardware for specific tasks, and engaging in informed discussions about computer performance and capabilities. For example, knowing the difference between RAM and storage is critical when deciding whether your computer is running slowly due to insufficient processing power or lack of storage space. Such knowledge translates into informed purchasing decisions and efficient problem-solving. Networking concepts are equally essential, and often misunderstood. Terms like "IP address," "DNS," "router," "firewall," and "bandwidth" define the structure and function of computer networks. An IP address uniquely identifies a device on a network, while DNS translates domain names (like google.com) into IP addresses. A router directs network traffic, while a firewall protects against unauthorized access, and bandwidth determines the capacity of the network to transmit data. These terms are fundamental to understanding how data flows across networks, both small home networks and vast internet infrastructures. For instance, understanding bandwidth limitations helps to troubleshoot slow internet speeds and make informed decisions about upgrading internet plans. Furthermore, a basic understanding of networking principles helps to identify and prevent potential security vulnerabilities, safeguarding personal data and mitigating risks.

Beyond these basics, numerous other specialized terms exist within each of these technology fields. "Agile development," "cloud computing," "machine learning," "database management systems," and "cybersecurity" are just a few examples of concepts that require understanding. Each represents a complex area of expertise, and mastering their associated jargon is essential for effective communication and collaboration within these fields. This means actively seeking out resources that explain these terms, engaging with others who are knowledgeable in these areas, and actively trying to integrate what you learn into your own work or projects. The continuous process of learning and practical application is key to mastering technical terminology. Learning these terms is not a passive activity; it's an active journey of expanding your knowledge and improving your understanding of increasingly complex systems. It's about building a contextual understanding that allows you to seamlessly integrate yourself into conversations and projects dealing with these essential components.

5.1 Software Development

Software development, at its core, is about problem-solving. You start with a need, perhaps a business need, a personal desire, or a societal problem, and you craft a solution using code. This might involve creating a website, designing a mobile app, or building a complex system for a large corporation. Every line of code is a small piece of that solution, a step towards making the digital world a more convenient and connected place. The skill lies not just in writing code but in understanding the bigger picture, the overall architecture and design principles.

Understanding programming languages is essential. Think of them as different dialects of the same digital tongue. Each language, like Python, Java, or C++, offers unique strengths and weaknesses, suited to different tasks and environments. Python, for instance, is known for its readability and versatility, making it popular for beginners and data science. Java, with its platform independence, is a mainstay in enterprise applications. Learning one language well builds a foundation that makes learning others easier, building upon the conceptual understanding of programming itself. Choosing your first language depends on your interests and goals; exploring different languages is crucial in understanding the landscape of software development.

Beyond the languages themselves lies the vast world of software development methodologies. Agile, Waterfall, Scrum—these are just a few of the frameworks used to structure and manage software projects. Agile, for instance, emphasizes iterative development and collaboration, allowing for flexibility and adaptation to changing requirements. Waterfall, a more traditional approach, follows a linear sequence of stages, with each stage completed before moving to the next. Choosing the right methodology is vital for efficient project management and successful outcomes. The most important element is not which methodology you use, but your ability to utilize its advantages while mitigating its limitations.

Then there's the importance of testing. No software is perfect on its first attempt; bugs are inevitable. Rigorous testing—unit testing, integration testing, system testing—is critical to ensuring that the software works as intended and is free of errors. It is not an afterthought, but an integral part of the development process. This includes automated testing, which greatly increases efficiency and helps identify and solve issues much earlier. Without robust testing, you risk delivering unstable and unreliable software. This can result in significant issues later on, especially if the problems are only discovered after release.

Finally, let's not forget the crucial role of collaboration. Software development is rarely a solo endeavor. Working effectively in a team, communicating clearly, and sharing knowledge are essential skills for success. Version control systems, like Git, are indispensable tools that allow teams to work together seamlessly, managing code changes and resolving conflicts. Even when you're working individually, sharing your code and getting feedback from others can drastically improve quality. Effective communication and collaboration ensure the success of not only the project, but also create a more enriching and rewarding experience for all involved. Understanding teamwork principles isn't just about technology, it's about human interaction and collaboration.

5.2 Computer Hardware

The central processing unit, or CPU, is the brain of your computer. Think of it as the conductor of an orchestra, directing the flow of information and processing instructions. Understanding its different components, like the cores and clock speed, is crucial for evaluating a computer's performance. More cores generally mean the computer can handle more tasks simultaneously, while a higher clock speed indicates faster processing of individual instructions. This is analogous to having more musicians in your orchestra versus each musician playing faster. A balance between both factors often yields the optimal performance. You need to consider your needs \item a graphic designer needs a different CPU than someone who primarily uses their computer for email. Random Access Memory (RAM) acts as your computer's short-term memory. It's where the data your computer is actively using resides, allowing for quick access. Imagine it as your desk—you keep the documents you're currently working on there for easy reach. Unlike long-term storage (hard drives or SSDs), RAM is volatile, meaning data is lost when the power is turned off. The more RAM you have, the more applications you can run simultaneously without experiencing slow-downs. Consider your workflow. If you consistently work with large files or multiple programs, then investing in more RAM is essential for a smooth user experience. Insufficient RAM leads to constant swapping of data between RAM and storage which drastically decreases performance.

Hard Disk Drives (HDDs) and Solid State Drives (SSDs) provide long-term storage for your files, operating system, and applications. Think of them as your filing cabinets. HDDs are mechanical devices with spinning platters, while SSDs utilize flash memory, making them significantly faster and more durable. SSDs are like having a well-organized, easily accessible filing cabinet, while HDDs can be likened to a sprawling, less organized archive. Choosing between them depends on your budget and priorities. SSDs provide a quicker boot time and faster application loading, while HDDs offer more storage capacity at a lower price point. The choice comes down to balancing speed and cost.

The graphics processing unit (GPU) is dedicated to handling visual computations, crucial for gaming, video editing, and other graphics-intensive tasks. It's like the visual effects team of your computer, handling the rendering of images and animations. A powerful GPU accelerates these processes, resulting in smoother gameplay or faster rendering times. The type of GPU you need depends heavily on your intended use. Casual users might not need a high-end GPU, while professional video editors or gamers will benefit from significantly more powerful

components. Do your research; it's important to pair a capable CPU and GPU for maximum benefit.
Motherboards act as the central communication hub connecting all the components within your computer, including the CPU, RAM, and storage devices. Consider it the building's electrical system. It facilitates the transfer of data between these components. Different motherboards support different CPUs and have varying expansion capabilities, including the number of RAM slots and expansion slots for additional cards. Choosing the correct motherboard is vital for compatibility; you must select a motherboard that works with your CPU socket type and your RAM requirements. It will determine what capabilities your build will have, such as extra ports or connections.
Power Supply Units (PSUs) provide the necessary electricity to power all of your components. Think of it as the power grid that feeds electricity to your computer. The wattage of the PSU determines its power capacity. A sufficient wattage is essential to ensure all your components are adequately powered without causing instability or damage. Underpowering your system can lead to sudden shutdowns and component failure. Choosing a PSU with enough wattage is crucial for system stability and longevity. Always check your individual component power requirements before purchase.
The case is the chassis that houses all your computer components. It's the physical structure that protects your delicate hardware from dust, damage, and physical impact. Different cases offer varying cooling options, expansion capabilities, and aesthetic designs. Choose a case with adequate airflow for optimal cooling performance, and ensure it has enough space for all your components. While aesthetics matter, prior-

itize features and functionality. Cooling solutions and available space will vary widely.

Understanding these fundamental computer hardware components and their functions is the first step in building or troubleshooting your computer system. It enables you to make informed decisions about what suits your needs and budget. Remember that your specific requirements will influence the choices you make, so it's crucial to identify your work style and needs before making any significant investment. Don't be afraid to seek assistance from online forums or professionals if you get stuck. This is merely an introduction, and there's a vast amount of additional information to discover.

5.3 Networking Concepts

Understanding computer networks requires grasping fundamental concepts, starting with the basic building blocks: nodes and links. Nodes represent any device connected to a network, from your laptop to a massive server; links are the pathways connecting these nodes, often represented by cables or wireless signals. Imagine a bustling city: the buildings are nodes, and the roads are links. This simple analogy helps visualize how data flows within a network, constantly moving between interconnected devices.

Network topologies define how these nodes and links are arranged. Common topologies include bus, star, ring, and mesh configurations. A bus topology resembles a single highway, all nodes connected to a single cable. A star topology, more common in modern networks, uses a central hub or switch, making it easier to manage and troubleshoot.

Think of a wheel; the hub is the center, and the spokes are the connections to each node. Ring and mesh topologies are more complex, offering redundancy and fault tolerance, critical in large-scale deployments but often less suitable for simpler home or small business setups. The best topology depends on the network's size and specific needs.

IP addresses are crucial for identifying devices on a network. They're like unique street addresses for each node, allowing data packets to reach the correct destination. These addresses consist of numerical identifiers, divided into IPv4 (32-bit addresses) and IPv6 (128-bit addresses), the latter designed to handle the rapidly growing number of connected devices. Understanding IP addresses is essential for configuring network settings, troubleshooting connectivity issues, and securing your network effectively against unauthorized access. Without unique IP addresses, network communication would be utterly chaotic. Subnets logically divide large networks into smaller, more manageable units, enhancing efficiency and security. Imagine dividing a large city into districts—this is precisely what subnetting accomplishes. It improves routing efficiency and security by controlling traffic flow. It also simplifies administration and allows for the assignment of IP addresses in a more organized manner, vital for larger networks with numerous devices. The concept of subnetting adds another layer to understanding the architecture and management of a network.

Network protocols govern how data is transmitted across networks. These are the sets of rules that allow devices to communicate efficiently. TCP/IP, a ubiquitous suite of protocols, underpins the internet. TCP ensures reliable data delivery, while IP handles addressing and routing. Understanding protocols like TCP and UDP (User Datagram Protocol) is crucial for comprehending how different applications utilize the network. TCP provides a reliable connection, ideal for applications like web browsing, whereas UDP prioritizes speed over reliability, suited for streaming applications.

Network security is paramount in today's interconnected world. Firewalls act as guardians, filtering incoming and outgoing network traffic, blocking malicious attempts. Intrusion detection systems (IDS) monitor network activity for suspicious patterns, alerting administrators to potential threats. Virtual Private Networks (VPNs) encrypt network traffic, ensuring secure communication over insecure networks. These tools are crucial in protecting against unauthorized access, data breaches, and other cyber threats. Implementing robust security measures protects your valuable data.

Understanding different types of networks is essential. Local Area Networks (LANs) connect devices within a limited geographical area, such as a home or office. Wide Area Networks (WANs) connect devices over a larger geographical area, such as the internet. Metropolitan Area Networks (MANs) bridge the gap between LANs and WANs, covering a city or region. These categorizations are based on their reach and the technology employed. Understanding this classification will help you effectively manage and apply your networking skills.

Finally, troubleshooting network issues requires systematic investigation. It starts with identifying the problem, whether it's slow connection speeds, connectivity issues, or data loss. Basic troubleshooting techniques involve checking cables, network settings, and device configurations. Using diagnostic tools can pinpoint the source of the problem more effectively. Troubleshooting isn't just about fixing problems;

it's about understanding the entire system and its underlying functions. The ability to systematically solve network issues is a valuable asset in any technical role.

6 Scientific Jargon

Understanding scientific jargon is crucial, especially for those working in interdisciplinary fields. It's a gateway to comprehending complex research papers, engaging in insightful discussions with scientists, and contributing effectively to collaborative projects. Mastering this specialized vocabulary isn't about memorizing a dictionary; it's about understanding the underlying concepts and how they're expressed.

Physics, for example, relies heavily on precise definitions. Terms like "quantum entanglement," "gravitational waves," and "string theory" might sound esoteric, but they represent rigorously defined concepts, backed by decades of experimentation and theoretical work. To grasp their meaning, delve into the core principles of quantum mechanics or general relativity. Don't just accept definitions at face value; understand their derivation and implications. Understanding the concepts behind the jargon allows you to use the jargon confidently and accurately, showing that you understand the subject matter and can effectively communicate with your peers.

Chemistry presents its own unique challenges. Consider the seemingly simple term "pH." It represents the concentration of hydrogen ions in a solution—a critical factor in countless chemical reactions and biological processes. Understanding pH involves grasping the logarithmic scale, the concept of acidity and alkalinity, and its practical implications in fields ranging from environmental science to medicine. Explore the concepts in detail and practice applying them. This means actively using the terms in your own thoughts and speech, rather than passively absorbing them. If you can explain a term clearly and simply to someone else, you've achieved a meaningful level of understanding.

However, simply memorizing definitions isn't enough. Effective comprehension requires understanding the relationships between terms and their broader context within the scientific framework. For example, knowing the definition of "enzyme" is only half the battle; true understanding emerges when you connect it to concepts like catalysis, active sites, and metabolic pathways. The more interconnections you make, the stronger your understanding becomes, making the seemingly complex jargon more accessible.

Furthermore, don't be afraid to ask for clarification. Scientists, like other professionals, often use jargon casually, sometimes without realizing it's unclear to others. Asking questions, whether it's during a lecture, a seminar, or in informal conversations with colleagues, demonstrates a genuine interest in learning and prevents misunderstandings. Moreover, don't hesitate to use resources like dictionaries, encyclopedias, and online learning platforms to enhance your vocabulary and deepen your understanding. This multi-faceted approach will reinforce the terms and their underlying significance.

The key to conquering scientific jargon is active learning. Don't simply read definitions passively; actively seek to understand the underlying concepts, explore the relationships between terms, and engage with the scientific community. Ask questions, challenge your understanding, and seek out additional resources. By adopting a proactive learning style and making a consistent effort to apply and expand upon what you learn, you will find that the daunting jargon becomes increasingly manageable and even meaningful. This journey will enhance not only your vocabulary but also your overall scientific comprehension, opening doors to further exploration and insightful discoveries. Scientific understanding grows through a deep grasp of the subject matter rather than superficial memorization of isolated words.

Consider the term "isomer." It seems simple enough – molecules with the same chemical formula but different structures. However, understanding the implications of isomerism requires knowledge of structural formulas, stereochemistry, and the impact of structural differences on chemical properties and biological activity. Similarly, consider "electrophoresis" – a technique with varied applications. Its understanding extends far beyond the definition; it also includes understanding the underlying principles of charge, electric fields, and the separation of molecules based on their properties. The significance of this lies not just in comprehending the basic definition, but in recognizing its applications across multiple scientific domains.

Effective communication hinges on accurately conveying and interpreting these intricate concepts. Therefore, proficiency with scientific jargon isn't merely about understanding individual terms; it's about using them correctly and applying them within appropriate contexts. This involves critically evaluating the precision of language used in scientific publications and presentations, thereby refining your own ability to communicate complex scientific information clearly and precisely.

Mastering this skill ultimately enhances scientific discourse and collaboration within the wider scientific community, leading to more efficient sharing of knowledge and advancement within the field.

Finally, remember that language evolves. New scientific discoveries constantly introduce novel terms and concepts, requiring continual learning and adaptation. This means staying updated on advancements in your field, actively seeking out relevant scientific literature, and participating in discussions with other experts. Engaging in this continuous learning process will ensure you remain proficient in the ever-evolving language of science, ensuring that you can confidently navigate the complexity of scientific jargon while actively contributing to the advancement of the field.

6.1 Physics Terms

Understanding the universe requires grappling with its unique language: physics. This chapter introduces fundamental concepts, focusing on clarity and practical application rather than overwhelming mathematical detail. We'll explore key terms, enabling you to better navigate scientific discussions and texts.

Newton's laws of motion, cornerstones of classical mechanics, describe the relationship between a body and the forces acting upon it. Inertia, the tendency of an object to resist changes in its state of motion, is crucial. A force, simply put, is an interaction that can alter an object's velocity. Newton's second law, F=ma (force equals mass times acceleration), quantifies this relationship—a larger force produces greater acceleration, all else being equal. Understanding these concepts is essential for grasping many physical phenomena, from the trajectory of a ball to the movement of planets.

Consider energy, a fundamental concept across physics. Kinetic energy, the energy of motion, depends on an object's mass and velocity. Potential energy, on the other hand, is stored energy, often due to position or configuration. For example, a ball held high above the ground possesses gravitational potential energy, which converts to kinetic energy as it falls. The conservation of energy, a fundamental principle, states that energy cannot be created or destroyed, only transformed from one form to another. This principle underpins many areas of physics, from thermodynamics to astrophysics. Mastering these energy concepts provides a solid foundation for understanding more complex topics.

Moving beyond mechanics, let's look at waves, ubiquitous in the physical world. A wave transfers energy without transferring matter. Think of ripples on a pond, sound waves traveling through air, or light waves traversing space. These waves possess characteristics such as wavelength (distance between successive crests), frequency (number of cycles per second), and amplitude (wave height). Understanding wave properties is crucial for understanding phenomena like sound, light, and even quantum mechanics. Many technologies, from radio to medical imaging, rely on manipulating and understanding wave behavior.

Electricity and magnetism are intrinsically linked, forming electromagnetism. Electric charge, a fundamental property of matter, comes in two forms: positive and negative. Like charges repel, while opposite charges attract. Electric current is the flow of electric charge. A magnetic field, invisible but powerful, surrounds any moving electric charge, influencing the behavior of other charged particles. Electromagnetism is central to numerous technologies, from generators and motors to communication systems and medical devices. Grasping these basic concepts opens the door to a deeper understanding of how electronics work.

Finally, let's touch on the concept of thermodynamics, dealing with heat and its relation to energy and work. Temperature, a measure of average kinetic energy of particles, is a crucial parameter. Heat, the transfer of thermal energy, flows from hotter to colder objects. The laws of thermodynamics govern energy transformations, particularly concerning efficiency and entropy, a measure of disorder in a system. Understanding thermodynamics is crucial in many applications, from designing engines to understanding biological processes. These laws are not just theoretical constructs; they have profound implications for engineering and technology. They determine the limits of energy conversion and efficiency in numerous systems.

In conclusion, this chapter presented a selection of fundamental physics terms, providing a starting point for those wanting to navigate the field's vocabulary. Understanding these terms – from Newton's laws to thermodynamics – offers a basis for exploring more advanced concepts. Remember, physics is a vast and intricate subject. But by focusing on these fundamental building blocks, and perhaps using a physics dictionary for further clarification, you can begin to decipher its rich vocabulary and appreciate the elegance and power of the underlying physical laws governing our universe. Further exploration will reveal even more intricacies and applications, enriching your understanding of the natural world. The journey into understanding the physical world begins with these core concepts, forming a crucial foundation for future learning.

6.2 Chemistry Terms

Atoms are the fundamental building blocks of all matter, incredibly tiny particles that combine to form molecules. Understanding this basic concept is crucial for navigating the world of chemistry. Molecules, in turn, are collections of two or more atoms bonded together, exhibiting unique properties distinct from their constituent atoms. Think of water (HO): two hydrogen atoms and one oxygen atom combine to create a liquid essential for life, vastly different from the individual gaseous elements.

The periodic table serves as a chemist's roadmap, organizing elements based on their atomic number and properties. Each element occupies a specific square, providing information such as its symbol, atomic mass, and electron configuration. This table is essential for predicting how elements will react with each other, forming the basis for understanding chemical reactions. Learning to navigate this table, recognizing patterns and trends among elements, is a fundamental skill for any aspiring chemist. Understanding the arrangement of elements, their valence electrons, and their reactivity allows you to predict the nature of chemical bonds and the resulting compounds.

Chemical bonding describes the forces that hold atoms together in molecules. There are several types of bonds, each with its own characteristics. Ionic bonds involve the transfer of electrons between atoms, creating ions with opposite charges that attract each other. Covalent bonds, on the other hand, involve the sharing of electrons between atoms, resulting in a stable molecule. Metallic bonds occur in metals and involve a sea of delocalized electrons shared among many atoms, giving rise to metals' characteristic properties like conductivity. Understanding the type of bond present in a molecule is crucial for understanding its properties, such as melting point, boiling point, and solubility.

Chemical reactions involve the rearrangement of atoms and molecules, resulting in the formation of new substances. These reactions can be represented using chemical equations, which show the reactants (starting materials) and products (resulting substances). Balancing these equations is crucial to ensure the conservation of mass during the reaction; the same number of each type of atom must be present on both sides of the equation. Stoichiometry is the study of the quantitative relationships between reactants and products in chemical reactions, providing a way to calculate the amount of product formed from a given amount of reactant. This is particularly relevant in industrial processes where precise control over reaction yield is crucial. Understanding stoichiometry is essential for accurate predictions of yields and efficient reaction design.

Acids and bases are fundamental chemical concepts with far-reaching implications. Acids donate protons (H ions), while bases accept protons. The pH scale measures the acidity or basicity of a solution, ranging from 0 (highly acidic) to 14 (highly basic), with 7 being neutral. Strong acids and bases completely dissociate in water, while weak acids and bases only partially dissociate. Understanding the pH scale is important in various contexts, from understanding biological systems to industrial processes. Many everyday substances, such as lemon juice (acidic) and baking soda (basic), demonstrate the properties of acids and bases. Accurate pH measurements are critical for many applications in medicine, environmental monitoring, and industrial chemical processing. The proper use of indicators can greatly assist in determining the pH of unknown solutions.

Organic chemistry deals specifically with carbon-containing compounds, the building blocks of life. Carbon's unique ability to form four bonds allows for the creation of a vast array of molecules with diverse structures and functions. Functional groups, specific arrangements of atoms within a molecule, determine the chemical properties of organic compounds. Understanding the properties and reactions of functional groups is crucial for comprehending the behavior of organic molecules. Organic chemistry also includes the study of hydrocarbons, which are composed only of carbon and hydrogen atoms, forming the basis for many fuels and materials. Alkanes, alkenes, and alkynes are just a few examples of hydrocarbon families. Learning the nomenclature and chemical reactions related to these compounds is critical to understanding many organic compounds.

Finally, understanding chemical nomenclature – the system for naming chemical compounds – is vital for effective communication within the field. There are systematic rules for naming inorganic and organic compounds, ensuring that chemists worldwide understand each other. Learning these rules, including the use of prefixes and suffixes to denote the number and types of atoms in a molecule, is an important step in mastering chemical terminology. The International Union of Pure and Applied Chemistry (IUPAC) establishes and standardizes these rules globally, promoting clear and consistent communication. This system simplifies the communication of complex molecular structures, avoiding ambiguity in research and industrial settings.

7 Conclusion: Mastering Jargon

Developing fluency in any specialized language requires consistent effort and a strategic approach. Don't expect overnight mastery; it's a gradual process of immersion and application. Think of it like learning a musical instrument—you wouldn't expect to play a concerto after a single lesson. Instead, focus on incremental progress, celebrating small victories along the way. Start with the basics, building a solid foundation before tackling more complex concepts. This systematic approach will significantly enhance your comprehension and retention. Remember, understanding the underlying principles of the field is crucial before tackling its specific jargon.

Active recall is far more effective than passive reading. After encountering a new term, try to define it in your own words without referring back to the source. This self-testing forces your brain to actively engage with the material, strengthening the neural pathways associated with that term. Create flashcards, use spaced repetition software, or simply test yourself regularly. The more you actively recall the definition, the better you'll retain it. This method isn't just about memorization; it's about building a deep understanding that translates into practical application. This differs significantly from merely passively reading a definition.

Context is everything. The same term can have different meanings depending on the field or even the specific situation. Pay close attention to the context in which a term is used. Analyze how the term functions within the sentences and paragraphs surrounding it. If you encounter an unfamiliar term, look for clues within the text to decipher its meaning. The surrounding information often provides valuable context to unravel the term's specific meaning. This contextual understanding is fundamental to truly mastering jargon. This is critical since a lack of contextual understanding leads to frequent misunderstandings.

Immerse yourself in the field. The best way to master jargon is through exposure. Read books, articles, and journals related to the specific field. Listen to podcasts and watch videos created by experts. Attend conferences and workshops. The more you are exposed to the language, the more familiar you'll become with it. This constant exposure is more effective than isolated study sessions. Consider it a full-body immersion into the world of specialized language, where understanding emerges naturally from regular engagement. This active engagement accelerates the learning process considerably.

Leverage online resources. There is a vast sea of information available online. Websites, online dictionaries, encyclopedias, and educational platforms are incredibly useful resources. Don't hesitate to use them to look up terms you don't understand. Many specialized websites offer explanations, examples, and additional context. Take full advantage of these free, readily accessible resources designed for learners like yourself. The effective use of these tools speeds up learning and solidifies understanding.

Don't be afraid to ask for help. If you're struggling with a particular term, don't hesitate to ask someone who is knowledgeable in the field for clarification. Experts often welcome the opportunity to share their knowledge and explain concepts in a clear and understandable way. Reaching out to professionals might even create networking opportunities, enriching your learning experience beyond just the jargon itself. Active engagement with professionals in the field proves immensely beneficial to mastery.

Jargon evolves continuously, reflecting advancements and shifts within each field. Staying updated requires ongoing effort. This continuous learning ensures you remain current with the changing language and its nuances. New terms arise, old terms become outdated, and meanings subtly evolve. This dynamic nature necessitates a continuous learning process to maintain proficiency. This constant adaptation keeps you at the forefront of the field's linguistic development.

Develop a personal glossary. As you encounter new terms, create your own personal glossary. Write down the term, its definition, and an example sentence illustrating its use. Regularly review your glossary to reinforce your understanding. This personalized approach enhances learning by actively engaging with the material. It's a far more effective technique compared to merely highlighting definitions in a textbook. This dynamic glossary evolves along with your understanding of the field.

7.1 Tips for Learning Jargon

Immerse yourself fully. Don't just passively read definitions; actively engage with the terms. Imagine yourself using the words in a conversation, writing a report, or giving a presentation. This active recall significantly strengthens memory retention. For example, if you're learning medical jargon, try describing a patient's symptoms using the new terms. Or, if you're grappling with legal language, draft a short contract incorporating the key phrases. This hands-on approach transforms passive learning into an active, engaging process, making jargon less intimidating and more readily accessible.

Context is king. Don't isolate jargon words; understand their meaning within their specific context. Each term carries nuances and subtleties that are only revealed through its application within its field. A single word can have vastly different meanings depending on the surrounding terms and the overall subject matter. This contextual understanding is crucial, because it's not just about memorization; it's about comprehension. Look for patterns and relationships between words, recognizing prefixes, suffixes, and root words that can help unlock the meanings of unfamiliar terms. This approach provides a structural understanding of jargon that extends beyond rote memorization. Consider joining online communities or forums where professionals in the field use jargon naturally. The context-rich environment facilitates a more rapid understanding, and interacting with peers naturally integrates the terms into your vocabulary.

Utilize diverse learning methods. Don't rely solely on reading. Experiment with various techniques that cater to different learning styles. Visual learners might find flashcards helpful, creating images or diagrams associated with specific terms. Auditory learners could benefit from recording themselves pronouncing the jargon, listening to podcasts, or attending webinars. Kinesthetic learners might find writing summaries or engaging in role-playing scenarios useful. The key is to find the most efficient learning path and adjust your approach as needed. Consider using mnemonics—memory aids like acronyms or rhymes—to help remember difficult or obscure terms. This technique taps into the creative side of learning, reinforcing retention through active engagement. Consistent, spaced repetition is another vital component. Reviewing material at increasing intervals helps embed the information in your long-term memory, transforming short-term retention into lasting comprehension.

Embrace resources strategically. Numerous resources can aid your jargon acquisition. Specialized dictionaries and glossaries provide precise definitions, contextual examples, and etymological origins. Online courses, tutorials, and webinars offer structured learning paths, often incorporating interactive elements that cater to diverse learning styles. Professional journals and industry publications provide authentic exposure to jargon in use, allowing you to contextualize your learning within the professional environment. Leverage these tools intelligently, recognizing that various resources cater to various learning styles and preferences. Remember that combining multiple resources often provides the most comprehensive and effective learning approach. For instance, using a glossary to define a term, then searching for its application in a professional journal, and finally discussing it within an online community. This multi-faceted engagement reinforces comprehension.

Cultivate consistent practice. The key to mastering jargon is consistent and deliberate practice. Actively seek opportunities to integrate the newly acquired terms into your everyday communication. When discussing topics related to your field, make a conscious effort to utilize the jargon appropriately. Don't be afraid to make mistakes; errors are valuable learning opportunities. Seek feedback from peers or mentors, who can provide corrections and guidance. This continuous immersion reinforces the language and allows you to recognize its nuances in a real-world context. The ultimate test of understanding lies in your ability to use jargon naturally and effectively, which only comes through persistent use and refinement. Make it a habit to review terms regularly, even after you believe you have mastered them. This helps solidify the information and ensures the knowledge remains readily available when needed. Incorporate the jargon into your personal notes, summaries, and presentations; this will subtly reinforce the information through repetitive engagement, subtly embedding it into your long-term memory.

7.2 Resources for Jargon

Dictionaries, specialized encyclopedias, and glossaries are your first line of defense. For medical jargon, Stedman's Medical Dictionary is a classic resource, offering comprehensive definitions and etymologies. Don't overlook online medical dictionaries; many offer detailed explanations, images, and even audio pronunciations, crucial for understanding complex terms like "thrombocytopenia" or "splenomegaly." For legal terms, Black's Law Dictionary remains the gold standard, its detailed entries providing not only definitions but also insightful historical context and usage examples. Explore online legal resources, such as those provided by law schools and legal organizations, which often include comprehensive glossaries and explanations of legal processes. The sheer volume of legal terminology can feel overwhelming; remember to focus on the areas most relevant to your needs.

Financial terminology often requires a nuanced understanding of economic principles. Investopedia provides a wealth of definitions and explanations, covering everything from basic concepts like "compound interest" to more complex topics such as "derivatives" and "hedge funds." Websites of reputable financial institutions often offer glossaries of their own terminology, providing context within specific financial products or services. Pay close attention to the context in which financial terms are used; a subtle shift in meaning can drastically alter the implications.

Navigating technical jargon requires a slightly different approach. For software development, sites like Stack Overflow offer not only definitions but also explanations, code examples, and community discussions. Understanding the nuances of programming languages like Python or Java requires delving into their official documentation; these often contain comprehensive glossaries and guides. For hardware and networking, sites specializing in technical support and reviews are invaluable. These sites often provide detailed explanations of components, protocols, and their interactions, making complex topics like network topology or processor architecture more manageable. Remember to cross-reference information from multiple sources to gain a well-rounded understanding.

Scientific jargon presents a unique challenge; the precision and complexity of scientific language demand careful study. For physics and chemistry terms, reputable university websites and online textbooks are essential. These resources not only provide concise definitions but also explain the underlying concepts, often with illustrative examples and diagrams. Scientific journals can be daunting, but scanning abstracts and key sections can provide exposure to specialized terminology within specific areas. Don't hesitate to utilize online resources to visualize abstract scientific concepts; simulations and interactive tools can greatly improve understanding.

Beyond specific field dictionaries and online resources, consider using language learning techniques. Flashcards can be extremely effective for memorizing new terms, especially when combined with spaced repetition systems. Active recall, where you try to define a term from memory before checking your answer, enhances retention. Building your own glossary tailored to your specific needs is a powerful strategy. Note down new terms, their definitions, examples of usage and any relevant diagrams or pictures. This self-created resource will not only enhance your understanding but also become a valuable reference for future use. Remember to review your glossary regularly to reinforce your learning.

Finally, don't underestimate the power of context. Immerse yourself in the field you're studying. Read articles, listen to podcasts, and watch videos related to the subject matter. The more you encounter specific terms in their natural context, the better you will understand their meaning and usage. Engage in conversations with professionals in the field, asking for clarification on unfamiliar terms. Networking and collaborative learning are invaluable in mastering specialized vocabulary. Remember, learning jargon is an ongoing process; embrace the challenge and enjoy the rewards of enhanced understanding and communication.

7.3 The Future of Jargon

The increasing interconnectedness of global communication, fueled by instantaneous digital exchange, presents a fascinating paradox for jargon. While specialized language remains crucial for efficient communication within niche fields, its future hinges on a delicate balance between precision and accessibility. We're moving away from a world where esoteric terms create impenetrable barriers. Consider the rise of citizen science initiatives; laypeople actively participate in research projects, necessitating clearer, more inclusive explanations of complex scientific concepts. This shift demands a conscious effort from experts to bridge the knowledge gap.

The future likely won't see the complete eradication of jargon; the nuanced terminology that efficiently conveys intricate ideas will remain. However, the way we use and understand it will transform significantly. Expect to witness a growing emphasis on plain language summaries alongside technical documentation. Imagine medical reports accompanied by concise, accessible patient summaries, or legal documents including layman's explanations of key clauses. This proactive approach facilitates better understanding and informed decision-making across all levels.

Technological advancements also play a critical role. Translation software, while still imperfect, continuously improves, potentially simplifying cross-disciplinary communication. Real-time language processing tools can identify and offer alternative, simpler phrasing for complex terms, making specialized content more widely accessible. Imagine software that automatically generates plain-language equivalents for legal jargon, allowing non-lawyers to grasp the essence of contracts and agreements.

Educational institutions will be instrumental in shaping the future of jargon. Curricula must emphasize not only the acquisition of specialized terminology but also the importance of clear, concise communication. Training professionals to translate their knowledge into language accessible to a wider audience will be paramount. Think of incorporating training modules into medical, legal, and financial education to specifically focus on simplifying complex language for diverse audiences.

The ethical implications are significant. Using jargon to obfuscate or exclude is increasingly unacceptable. Transparency and accessibility are crucial, especially in fields dealing with public health, legal rights, and financial literacy. Over-reliance on jargon can lead to misinformation and unequal access to information. For example, overly technical medical explanations can create anxiety and mistrust, while unclear financial terms can lead to poor financial decisions. We must strive for a future where jargon's utility is balanced with a commitment to equitable understanding.

Furthermore, the future of jargon involves a deeper understanding of the audience. Effective communication means adapting the language to the specific knowledge level and needs of the recipient. Instead of assuming a shared understanding of technical terms, professionals must actively assess their audience's background and tailor their communication accordingly. This includes considering cultural contexts and language barriers. This nuanced approach necessitates ongoing dialogue and feedback, ensuring that jargon doesn't inadvertently marginalize certain groups.

Looking ahead, the future of jargon is not about elimination, but evolution. It's about harnessing the power of specialized language while ensuring it doesn't become a barrier to communication. This requires a collective effort from professionals, educators, and technologists to promote clear, concise, and accessible language across all fields. The goal is not to eliminate jargon entirely, but to make it a tool that promotes understanding and collaboration rather than confusion and exclusion. The success of this transformation depends on our collective commitment to responsible language use and a future where knowledge is shared effectively and equitably. The proactive approach to clear communication will be the hallmark of future professional discourse. This careful consideration of audience and context will be key to unlocking the full potential of professional collaboration.

www.ingramcontent.com/pod-product-compliance
Lightning Source LLC
LaVergne TN
LVHW022022200926
848481LV00007B/2491